CURE SLEEP
APNEA

Cure Sleep Apnea

Everything About Sleep Apnea
And Sleep Apnea Treatment

Ray Smith

TABLE OF CONTENT

About Sleep Apnea

Imagine yourself in deep sleep. Suddenly, you find yourself feeling hard to breathe. You feel as if you totally can't breathe or that your breathing is extremely shallow. Scary? Definitely is!

This condition is commonly known as sleep apnea. This temporary breathing stop could last from a few seconds to a few minutes. It could happen many times in the span of a single hour. Sometimes, more than twenty times in a single sixty minute span. It is definitely a very difficult condition to have.

However, you will feel that your breathing becomes much easier after that. This would be accompanied by snorting and choking. Without a doubt, this condition would heavily affect the quality of sleep at night. You would have trouble getting enough sleep. During the day, you would feel extremely tired and sleepy.

Another thing that makes sleep apnea difficult is the fact that sleep apnea is hard to be diagnosed. You can't just detect sleep apnea with a regular exam with your doctor. As this condition happens when you are soundly asleep, you may not even realize that you have it until someone tells you about this.

It could be a spouse or other people who share a room with you. Even if they were to realize something weird with your sleeping, it doesn't mean that they realize that you are having a sleep apnea condition.

There are millions of people suffering from sleep apnea but have no idea about it. Most of them tend to be overweight and this condition normally affects more man than women. Your age could also heavily affect your possibility of having it. The older you are, the higher the possibility of having it. For women, the chances of them getting sleep apnea gets higher when they reach the post-menopausal stage.

According to a research done, minority groups like Hispanics and Pacific Islanders have a higher possibility of developing sleep apnea compared to other ethnic groups. Besides that, sleep apnea could also be inherited from genes.

You would also have a higher possibility of developing this condition if you have small airways in your nose, throat and mouth. Younger children who have larger tonsil tissues than the general norm would also develop sleep apnea.

There are also higher risks of developing sleep apnea if you have several other symptoms or bad habits. Smokers are known to have a higher chance. Those who have a high blood pressure, heart failure previously or stroke-potential patients have a higher risk of sleep apnea as well.

Without a doubt, sleep apnea is a condition that could affect many groups of people. In the next chapter, we would discover how your weight affects the quality of your sleep. This is important as your weight plays a very important role in developing sleep apnea.

Your Weight Affects Your Sleep

As explained in a previous chapter, sleep apnea happens when you stop breathing or have shallow breaths for a moment during your sleep. Medical terminology defined this condition as when an individual literally stops breathing for a few moments. Generally, there are two types of sleep apnea - Central Sleep Apnea and Obstructive Sleep Apnea.

Sleep apnea is a condition which is extremely common among those who are morbidly obese. Some people would even find it necessary to wear an oxygen mask to ensure they get to breathe properly should an emergency emerges.

This happens because their weight bares down on their chest and crushes their lungs and rib cage. According to medical research, this situation is most common among middle-aged men who are overweight.

This is a very scary situation for those people who are close to you. Those people who have sleep apnea would go through a period where people feel like they aren't going to wake up. This becomes very life-threatening for the sufferer and needs to be dealt with.

Those who are morbidly obese would commonly deal with episodes of difficult breathing over their lifetime. They would commonly have a great problem with snoring and they would constantly gasp for air. With obstructive sleep apnea, it would pose a great danger for your heart because your body finds it hard to obtain air from your difficult breathing. The deprivation of oxygen stops the blood from flowing well around the body.

Those who are diagnosed with sleep apnea also have certain symptoms such as feeling irritable, moodiness, headaches, decreased sexual drive, increased heart rate, depression and anxiety. There are many symptoms of sleep apnea and they would affect people in different ways.

There is also a correlation between congenital and congestive heart failure with sleep apnea. Like all symptoms, these is also most commonly among those who are morbidly obese and have excess weight in them. This is very severe and the individual may not have treated the condition for a long period. As such, the condition may be no longer treatable.

According to another research, those who are Down's Syndrome are more likely to develop obstructive sleep apnea. This is because those who are with Down's Syndrome are more likely to develop an enlarged head, tonsils, tongues and narrowing of the nasopharnyx.

Medical procedures could also cause sleep apnea. Pharyngeal flap surgery is known to cause sleep apnea because after the surgery, it would affect the breathing pattern. If not monitored, it could be very life threatening.

Doctors and ENT (Ear, Nose and Throat) specialists propose different treatments when dealing with sleep apnea. They would take into account the severity of your condition and plan a form of treatment for those diagnosed with condition.

Among the factors that need to be considered include:

- Severity Of Sleep Apnea
- Individual Medical History
- Cause Of Sleep Apnea Obstruction

The specialists would propose treatments such as a total lifestyle change; avoid certain food and taking medications that help relax your nervous system.

If you are someone who is severely obese, losing weight is most important. You may also need to quit smoking and create other sleeping changes. This may include sleeping on a slanted pillow or sleeping on a special bed.

However, the most important is to start your weight loss. Don't make it a habit to sleep for too long hours as being active is the way to ensure that you lose weight. I have seen situations where people lose around forty pounds in a few months and their sleep apnea condition improves drastically. However, a total lifestyle change is also needed. This may include a total change in eating habits.

Such lifestyle change helps to maintain your weight. From here, they are able to get other forms of treatment which would further enhance their ability to cope with sleep apnea.

This may include getting a gastric bypass, which is a surgery that helps divide the stomach into a small upper pouch and a lower pouch. It would also rearrange the intestines to ensure that your breathing becomes easier.

Another common surgery is a lap band. This is a reversible surgery but to maintain your weight loss, a lifestyle change is still needed. Generally speaking a lap band surgery is a surgery which helps make the stomach smaller, thus helping with the weight loss. You would get full faster and thus eat lesser.

Fatality Of Sleep Apnea

From the previous chapters, it is clear that sleep apnea is a very serious sleep disorder that could threaten your life and at many times, very fatal. Those who suffer from sleep apnea sleep very normally, but their ability to breathe would be block the moment they are asleep.

This inability to breathe comes from the over-relaxed muscles in the throat. As such the muscles would collapse into the airway. From here, the body sends a signal to your brain that the breathing has been blocked as causes the person to wake up to breathe normally again.

Such interrupted breathing would occur many times throughout the night. It could occur up to fifty times in a single hour, although most of it last for just a few seconds. Very often, someone who suffers from this disorder isn't even aware that they are suffering from this. They have no idea why they feel tired during the day.

Obstructive sleep apnea is the most common form of sleep disorder. Some sufferers would also suffer from Central sleep apnea as well. This condition is commonly known as mixed sleep apnea.

Obstructive sleep apnea affects 15% to 20% of adults. If left untreated, this sleep disorder would be extremely life-threatening and be fatal. This condition is also an underlying cause of other illness like heart disease, pulmonary hypertension, stroke and systemic hypertension.

To cure sleep apnea, there are several forms of treatment. They are surgical and noninvasive. When someone is first diagnosed with sleep apnea, the first line of therapy to control sleep apnea is to use this treatment known as positive airway pressure (PAP).

This is a noninvasive form of treatment. In this form of treatment, a machine would deliver a constant flow of air through a mask which is worn while in deep sleep. A sleep technician would determine the force of the air flow. This is determined through a sleep study, delivered overnight.

To treat a milder to moderate case, dental devices are also used to treat sleep apnea. There are two categories of dental devices - mandibular or advancing devices. Mandibular devices are more commonly used. They are normally attached to your upper jaw and helps pull the lower jaw with the base of the tongue forward. This helps improve the airflow.

For most people with sleep apnea, medications are not very helpful. However, some of them still take antidepressants or mondafinal to control the symptoms that they would face.

The PAP machine is used together with supplemental oxygen. Be clear that oxygen can't prevent the airway collapse or sleep fragmentation. However, oxygen is still important because it prevents the drop of blood oxygen levels when your airway collapses.

Besides all this, there is also surgery that would help cure obstructive sleep apnea. This may include palatal implants, corrective jaw surgery and tracheostomy. From this surgery, their quality of life would generally change for the better.

Three Types Of Sleep Apnea

Generally speaking, there are three categories of sleep apnea. However, only two categories are most commonly talked about. The most common form of sleep apnea is obstructive sleep apnea. For this kind of sleep apnea, your throat muscles would collapse while you're asleep.

The other more common form of sleep apnea is called central sleep apnea. This condition happens when your breathing muscles isn't receiving the right signals. The most uncommon one, mixed sleep apnea, is a combination of the two.

In this chapter, we would go into more details about all three different types of sleep apnea. From here, you would better understand what specific sleep apnea that you have. This would allow you to be clearer about your condition.

Obstructive Sleep Apnea

Obstructive Sleep Apnea (OSA) blocks the airways in your throat. Among the other things that happen when you have this form of sleep disorder include:

- Throats muscles collapse inwards while you are deep asleep and you're having difficulties breathing.

- Air would go through the upper airway. The upper airway includes your throat, mouth and nose areas.
- Your muscles would get wider and they block the collapse to ensure that the airway is open.
- Your blood would have less oxygen and your lungs would need to absorb air from the outside.
- Sleep apnea happens when the tissues at the back of your throat are blocked temporarily. You would stop breathing for a moment and would need to wake up to gasp for breath.
- You may not even wake up, even if you have trouble breathing and make snorting sounds.

When you have more than five apnea episodes an hour, you are considered to have obstructive sleep apnea.

Central Sleep Apnea

Central Sleep Apnea (CSA) isn't as common as Obstructive Sleep Apnea. This form of sleep disorder starts from the brain, which operates as a central nervous system. Your brain would not send the right signal to the airway muscles to ensure that your breathing is alright.

The oxygen levels in your body decreases and you would wake up. However, you won't wake up every time, just most of the time.

There is also another method to determine if you have this condition. If you have heart failure or heart disease, you are most probably experiencing CSA.

Complex or Mixed Apnea

As mentioned earlier in this book, Complex or Mixed Sleep Apnea is a combination of both OSA and CSA. When diagnosed with this form of sleep apnea, the main condition that you need to face is Obstructive Sleep Apnea.

Additionally, because of the pressure from the airways, you would also have constant Central Sleep Apnea as well. If you use Continuous Positive Airway Pressure (CPAP), you would be able to acknowledge Central Sleep Apnea. This normally happens when the obstruction has been cleared.

Symptoms Of Sleep Apnea

Perhaps the most obvious symptoms of having sleep apnea is the constant snoring which is loud and consistent. You may pause snoring for a moment but you may also choke or gasp after pausing.

When sleeping on your back, the snoring would get louder while it wouldn't be as loud if you sleep on your sides. The snoring may not be every night but it may increase and get louder as you sleep.

When you are sleeping while snoring, you would have no idea that you have such breathing issues. You may only notice it when other people notice you. Other people would see the signs while seeing you asleep and will tell you if they become a pattern, which is if they are aware. However, just because you are a chronic snorer, it doesn't necessarily mean that you have sleep apnea.

One main sign that you have sleep apnea is that you have trouble keeping awake during the day. You would feel disengaged with your daily activities and may find yourself falling asleep constantly.

The moment you are not doing anything, you may fall asleep easily. You may also put yourself in certain accidents. When you fall asleep while driving or working, it increases your chances of accidents.

Besides that, other common symptoms of sleep apnea also include:

- Frequent urinations late in the day
- Morning headaches
- Feeling moody or experiencing a change in your personality
- Struggling to concentrate or focus
- Feeling dry throat in the morning when you wake up

The muscles in your throat are important in keeping the airways open to ensure that air would get into your lungs. However, those who suffer from sleep apnea would find that their throat muscles are relaxed. As such, your airway are blocked and your lungs with be devoid of air.

Those who have Obstructive Sleep Apnea also experience certain additional symptoms such as:

- Those who have a tiny head and neck would have a problem because the size of the airway is smaller in your mouth and throat.
- Your muscles in your throat and the tongue would be more relaxed that should be.
- If you are overweight, you would have extra soft fat tissue. As such, the tissue would get thick at the windpipe. There isn't too much of an opening for the airways.
- As an older adult, your brain signals nay not keep your throat muscles stiff like they should.

- When your airways are blocked, you would end up snoring loudly when you are asleep.

Besides all this, your low oxygen levels may make you difficult to have a good night's sleep. Your upper airway muscles get tight and your windpipe is open. You may be able to breathe normally again until you start choking or snorting.

Together with the low levels of oxygen and insufficient sleep, your stress hormones are released. This would increase the possibility of you having high blood pressure, heart attack, abnormal heartbeats and a stroke.

Besides that, these hormones could also cause a heart failure in you. If left untreated, you could also develop obesity and diabetes.

Diagnosing Sleep Apnea

Most of the time, physicians diagnose sleep apnea based on family and medical histories. It is the main factor when they are in this diagnosis although they would also conduct a physical examination.

This examination would study the symptoms that you have. If the signs, patterns and symptoms are similar to the common symptoms, then they would ask you for a sleep study.

A sleep study is a test done to measure your sleeping patterns. From here, they would determine the quality and quantity of your sleep. The studies would show the problems with your sleep. If you are indeed partially diagnosed and need to have a sleep study, you should definitely get one.

This study determines if you are diagnosed with a sleep disorder like sleep apnea. This has very important consequences. You need to understand if you have a sleep disorder as it can has dire consequences for your health.

Those professionals who are experienced in sleep studies could easily diagnose a sleep apnea condition. They would then provide the appropriate treatment so you could sleep better during the night.

You should be extremely honest to the professional physician so that he or she would be clear about any adverse sleeping habits that you have.

Common adverse sleeping habits include fatigue and sleepiness throughout the day. You also need to tell the physician if you have difficulties sleeping or waking up constantly in the middle of the night. You may even be suffering from sleep disorders that you aren't aware of.

You physician would also research more about your condition. They would need to analyze your sleeping schedule or ask your close family members about any chronic snoring they experience while you are deep asleep.

The physicians who are experienced with dealing with sleep disorders are known as sleep specialists. They could easily diagnose and provide the appropriate treatment for anyone with sleep disorder.

Many professionals also recommend creating and keeping a sleep diary for a few weeks. Two week, preferably. This helps the sleep study. Common things to include in your sleep diary include:

- What time you went to bed
- What time you woke up
- How many hours did you sleep
- How many times you woke up at night
- How long it took for you to fall asleep
- Do you take any medication the previous night
- Were you wide awake when you wake up in the morning

- Were you tired when you wake up in the morning
- Were you sleepy in the morning
- Did you consume any caffeine during the day
- Did you consume any alcohol during the day
- Did you have any naps during the day
- The length of your naps
- Were you sleepy or tired during the day
- Were you alert or wide awake during the day

Some of these questions may be extremely difficult for you to answer. It is understandable, but try your best to answer them. This discipline would go a long way towards understanding your sleeping condition. To understand better your condition, the sleep professional may also ask about the following:

- Do you snort while sleeping
- Do you experience any gasping for air during sleep
- Do you experience any morning headaches

From the results of the diary, you would determine a few things. If you put in the discipline, you would better discover if you have frequent naps throughout the day, the number of times you wake up at night, how long it takes to sleep and whether you are awake during the day.

All these would better help your physician determine your condition.

Physical Exams For Sleep Apnea

During the physical examination performed by your physician, he would check your nose, mouth and throats. The physician would be on the lookout for extra or enlarged tissues.

Children who have sleep apnea would normally have an enlarged tonsil. After a physical checkup and the physician is clear that the patient do indeed have an enlarged tonsil, a diagnosis isn't even necessary. He would just need to check out the medical history.

Meanwhile, the diagnosis for adults is slightly different. The physician would look for an enlarged uvula. It is a piece of tissue which sits and hangs from the back of your mouth. The physician would also be on the lookout for a soft palate. Your palate is located at the back of your throats and is commonly known as the roof of your mouth.

Family Members Help To Detect Sleep Apnea

As most people have no idea that they suffer from sleep apnea, having someone close to you to determine sleep abnormalities while you are asleep would help. The sufferer has no idea that their breathing is affected during their sleep. Besides, they don't even take into seriousness when someone tells them that they are a chronic snorer.

A family member can help them in various ways include:

- Bring into their awareness of their chronic snoring
- Advise them to seek a physician
- Be there for them. Support them emotionally. It could be a very testing

time for them and they need all the support they need

- If they are confirmed diagnosed with sleep apnea, advise them to be strict with the instructions. This may also include a total change in their lifestyle.

Diagnose Sleep Apnea With Sleep Studies

To perform sleep study, it is normally conducted in a sleep center or sleep lap. It may or may not be in a hospital. Depending on the physician, you may have an overnight stay to further diagnose your sleep situation.

Perhaps the best thing about sleep study is the fact that you won't need to endure any pain. Only problem that some people would face is the skin irritation as a result from the sensors used. However, the moment the sensors are removed, you wouldn't feel them anymore.

If the study is done during the day, you can bring a book to prevent you from boredom. There are no risks when doing this sleep study but it takes several hours.

The most common form of sleep study is called the polysomnogram (PSG Test). It is conducted in a sleep center and would require an overnight stay. For this test, you would have electrodes and monitors on different parts of your body.

This ranges from your face, chest, scalp, fingers and limbs. While you are sleeping the physician monitor different things including brain activity, muscle activity, eye movement, heart rate and rhythm, blood pressure and oxygen levels in your blood.

These are all important indication in your diagnosis.

When you sleep, the physician would use sensors to check on your condition. After the PSG test, the sleep specialist would go through the result to further understand your condition. They may be able to determine if you truly have sleep apnea and the severity of your condition. From here, they are able to chart a course of treatment.

Another common test, the Multiple Sleep Latency Test (MSLT), determines how sleepy you are during the day. It is performed after you are tested for PSG. They will place devices on your scalp to monitor your condition.

This test requires you to take a nap of a minimum of five times a day, ranging from around twenty minutes for each. This is done in two hours gap throughout the day to ensure your alertness.

The testers would check how long it takes for you to get to sleep and the length in which you nap. People who take less than five minutes to get to sleep are commonly known to be higher risk of having sleep disorder.

When the tests are finished, the sleep specialist would provide the appropriate report together with a detailed treatment option.

Find A Sleep Specialist

There are several organizations which help you find a qualified sleep specialist. They include:

- American Academy of Dental Sleep Medicine (AADSM)
- American Board of Sleep Medicine (ABSM)
- American Academy of Sleep Medicine (AASM)

They are made up of different groups of professionals from physicians, researchers and dentists. They work with people of different conditions and are affected with sleep apnea in various degrees. They are important people who help the advancement of sleep medication and research.

Physicians and researchers who serve on related boards are commonly known as 'board certified' in the sleep medication specialty. ABSM provides a constant updated listing of sleep specialists you can find locally.

They split them up into the state they are in, for your convenience. AADSM, meanwhile, have an updated listing of dentists who specialize in sleep apnea treatment.

Search for their website to have an updated listing of the professionals you can find. This would go a long way towards improving your sleep condition.

Children Who Have Sleep Apnea

Hyperactive and aggressiveness are among the main symptoms when a child is diagnosed with sleep apnea. As such, it would greatly affect their studies and their social life with other children.

At times, their sleep would be greatly disturbed and they may even wet the bed. During the day, some children may even breathe using their mouth instead of their nose.

As with the adults, children suffer the almost the same symptoms as well. Among them include loud snoring, gasping for air, snorting and temporary breathing stoppage. These are all similar to what adults' experience.

However, sleep apnea in children can't always be detected. Many physicians would just assume that what the children is facing is merely hyperactive-ness. They may feel that it's not a big deal. You have to be vary about it if you feel there's a possibility of your child having this condition.

There are several things you could do if you want to find out if your child has sleep apnea. Among them include:

- Consult a ENT (Ear, Nose, Throat) Specialist

- Discuss about the possibility of sleep apnea with your child's pediatrician and tell them about the condition of your child.
- Seek help from a pulmonologist who specializes in children. A pulmonologist is a lung specialist.
- Consult other professionals such as psychiatrists, psychologists or other medical professionals.

Be sure to check if your health insurance covers for such consultation, if you have one. You would be able to save a lot of money from here.

If upon further discussion and the medical professional feels that there is a need for further testing, check if the physician is qualified to treat children with sleep apnea. They need to be board qualified and don't be afraid to ask for their credentials. You need someone qualified to do this as this is your child's health. For something as delicate as this, you need someone capable to deal with care and attentiveness.

In this process, you need to be very honest with your physician and tell him if your child is taking any medication. You also need to bring to his awareness any allergy that your child might have. These are all medical considerations that your doctor would have to make.

Besides that, you should also share with them any behavioral or developmental issues that the child has. The information of their sleeping patterns and their naps are also valuable information for the doctor's diagnosis.

Like adults, the child may also need to take a sleep study or perform a PSG test to determine their condition. To determine the severity of their condition, other tests might even be done. Among them include:

- Electrocardiogram (EKG) - Used to determine the heart rate and rhythm measurement.
- Electroencephalogram (EEG) - Used to measure brain waves.
- Electroculogram (EOG) - Used to measure chin and eye
- Chest Bands Testing - To determine breathing movement measurements
- Monitor Testing - Determine levels of oxygen and carbon dioxide in the child's blood.

Most of the sleep study for children would require a stay at the sleep center. However, it should be noted that they aren't many such centers which specialized in sleep apnea for children. If you can't find for one such center, you can seek a center used for adults one. They are similar as the machines used could be used for children as well.

You would need to check with them first about this. Take time to call up the facility to find out if they could work with children with sleep apnea. Similar to adults, you would need to seek out various groups to determine if they are qualified sleep specialist. Such things are very important.

If you find your child having sleep apnea, you need to treat them immediately. Like with adults, if sleep apnea isn't treated immediately, there is potential to experience serious health issues.

It won't only affect their health. It would also affect their studies, self-esteem and relationships with others. Don't take for granted that they are going through a tough period. If there is a possibility of sleep apnea, seek help straight away.

Sleep Apnea Treatments

The main purpose of treating sleep apnea is so that the sufferer could breathe regularly during their sleep. This is primarily focused on Obstructive Sleep Apnea. From this treatment, the patient would be relieved from the loud snoring and being chronically sleepy during daytime.

Sleep apnea treatment would also reduce the possibility of other medical problems like heart disease, high blood pressure and diabetes. To deal with sleep apnea, there are

several treatments to consider. Among them
include:

- Make A Lifestyle Change
- Surgical Procedures
- Continuous Positive Airway Pressure
  (CPAP)
- Sleep Apnea Pillows

Such treatments can be used together. After
the right treatment, you would get more sleep
during the night and be more energized
during the day. Your health would be better
and you feel happier as your emotions won't
be affected by the constant sleep interruptions
at night.

You not only will help yourself, but your
partner would benefit from it too. He or she
would be able to get more quality sleep as you

wouldn't be disturbing throughout the night with your loud snoring and snorting.

Make A Lifestyle Change

Those who sleep on their back are generally more prone to developing sleep apnea. How you position yourself when you lie down on bed can be the thing that affects your sleep. It determines the number of times you experience sleep apnea during the night and the severity of it.

Obstructive sleep apnea has also to do with gravity. This situation causes your throat to not get sufficient airflow while you are lying on your back. Those who sleep on their back could experience more than seventy sleep apneas in a single hour.

To get rid of this situation, it is advisable to change. You should sleep on your left of right side. However, this advice may not help those people who are overweight. Therefore a complete lifestyle change is required. Among the change include:

- **Lose Weight.** If you are overweight, you need to lose weight. When we have excess weight, our throats are blocked. Losing weight would help your throat be less restrictive. Try consuming more healthy food like fruits or vegetables.

- **Exercise Regularly.** Regular exercise would help you lose weight and keep your airflow natural throughout the body. If you are not sure about what sort of exercises to perform, talk to your physician.

- **Stop Taking Any Sort Of Medications.** Don't take sleeping pills or any other medication unless you really need it. They don't help you over the long term. Don't depend on alcohol as a sedative to make you sleep.

- **Use A Nasal Spray or Stick.** If you have trouble keeping your nasal area opened, you should use a nasal spray or stick. The nasal area's passageway should be open and not blocked. Try decongestants if you want, although it is just for short term use.

- **Change Your Sleeping Methods.** For those who normally sleep on their back, it could be a huge task for them to change the way they sleep. Try sleeping on the side or on your stomach. The reason why sleeping on your back isn't recommended is because the soft palate of your throat and tongue would sit on the back. This situation creates a blockage in the airway.

- ***Elevate Your Head.*** Try inserting a soft pillow around the neck to ensure that your head would be able to take in more oxygen.
- ***Stop Smoking.*** Smoking is perhaps the one thing that you should stop right away regardless of the condition you are in. Smoking makes your sleep apnea condition worst as if affects your airflow.

You may also want to try other alternative medication like acupuncture. Although there isn't any research to support the use of acupuncture as a valid tool to cure sleep apnea, there have been results to prove its effectiveness.

However, it would be better if you first seek the advice of your physician before using any alternative treatment to cure sleep apnea. If a mere lifestyle change isn't sufficient for you to cure sleep apnea, you condition may be more serious than the norm. Therefore, you need to seek out other forms of treatment.

Surgical Procedures

Another treatment option to consider is surgery. After the right surgical procedure, the excess tissue removed from your nose or throat would help you breathe better.

Such procedure is performed only in a specialized hospital. You could also look for surgery which stiffen or shrink excess tissue. From here, your lower jaw would also be reset.

If you decide to perform the shrinking procedure, you need to get some shots into your tissue area. If the tissue excess are shrunk more, you would probably need other treatments besides the shot.

The stiffening process includes creating a small cut in the excess tissue and place a small piece of stiff plastic. Ask your doctor for further clarification if you want to understand this process better.

Pre-surgery, the doctor would give you some medication to ensure that you are asleep. This ensures that you wouldn't feel anything during the procedure. When this surgery is performed, you would experience certain pain in your throat for around a week or two.

Among the other forms of surgical procedures to treat sleep apnea includes:

(1) Tracheostomy Surgery

If previous surgical treatments didn't help you, you should look to perform this surgery. It also helps if your sleep apnea is so severe that it is life threatening.

The doctor would make an opening in your neck and a tube made of either metal or plastic is inserted. This helps you breathe. This opening is covered during the daytime and uncovered at night while you are asleep. Air should come in and out of your lungs while you sleep.

(2) Unulopalatopharyngoplasty Procedure (UPPP)

UPPP is a procedure where tissue is taken from the back of your mouth. From the top portion of your throat, tissue is removed. In certain situations, your tonsils and adenoids are removed as well.

Your snoring would stop after performing this surgery. However, it needs to be noted that there would still be tissue located further down your throat. As such, it is unlikely to treat your sleep apnea. While there are tissues still in there, your air passage wouldn't open. For UPPP, you need to go to a hospital to perform it.

This surgery is also extremely painful and it would take several weeks for you to recover. This condition is normally performed only on those who have very severe obstructive sleep apnea.

This isn't one of those surgeries that you can get and then your life would return to normal straight away. Among the complications that may arise from UPPP include:

- Problems with swallowing
- Finding it hard to smell
- Soft palate and throat unable to work properly

- Infected throat, if antibiotics are not given before surgery
- Fluids come up from your mouth and nose

(3) Maxillomandibular Procedure

This procedure is done to prevent any throat obstruction. This is done by making the space between your soft palate and tongue larger.

The upper and lower portion of your jaw is moved to the front and this is how the enlargement is created. It is a complex procedure and you may need an orthodontist and an oral surgeon to perform it simultaneously.

The surgeon would use laser to remove unnecessary tissues at the back of your throat. Besides that, they could also use radiofrequency energy. Both of them are extremely effective in relieving snoring but they can't be dependent to solely treat obstructive sleep apnea.

Besides that, there are other procedures that you can use to fix your snoring. Some could help with sleep apnea treatment. Bear in mind however that such procedures are not permanent cures for this disorder. They include:

- Nasal Surgery
- Get Rid of enlarged tonsils

Other surgery can also be used to deal with possible abnormalities on your face. Besides that, surgery can also deal with other forms of obstructions which cause sleep apnea. Some are done individually while some can be performed together.

Other common surgery includes:

- Plastic surgery on your chin
- Hyoid surgery, where the bone under your chin is moved towards the front. This moves the tongue muscles.
- Tongue advancement - A surgery which involves cutting the intersection between the jawbone and the tongue.

You have to be clear that surgery to treat sleep apnea isn't a guarantee.

If you experience Central Sleep Apnea, there are different therapies to be used. They may include.

- Continuous Positive Airway Pressure (CPAP)
- Bilevel Positive Airway Pressure (BiPAP) - A procedure where higher pressure is used to ensure that you can inhale better.

During the exhale, your air pressure would be lower and this helps strengthen your breathing if you have central sleep apnea. It is a powerful device that automatically detects if you haven't been breathing properly after a few seconds.

- Adaptive Servo-Ventilation (ASV) - A form of airflow device that feels how you normally breath and keeps your information in a computer. When you are deep asleep, ASV works to ensure that you have a normal breathing pattern and remove any breathing pauses. This procedure is better that CPAP if you have central sleep apnea.

Surgery for sleep apnea isn't a guarantee. You would still have possible recurrence of sleep apnea. Using any sort of surgery won't cure your condition right away. You need to do more than that.

Continuous Positive Airway Pressure (CPAP)

Continuous Positive Airway Pressure (CPAP) is one of the main methods in dealing with sleep apnea. It is a method where the machine produces air pressure with a mask. To receive the air, you wear the mask and it is situated on your nose while asleep.

When using CPAP, you get more air pressure compared to just breathing normally with the air from the outside. The air pressure from the machine would ensure that the passageways in your upper airways are open. It would prevent snoring and sleep apnea over the long term. When you are first starting to use this machine, it is normal to feel uncomfortable with it. You may not feel right at first but with the right adjustments, you would get used to it.

If you find your mask hard to settle in, you may need to find another one that suits you. You could also use a humidifier together with a CPAP to ensure extra comfort. You may also have other problems if you use it. However, persist along it. The problems are just temporary. If the discomfort lasts, talk to your physician about it so that he could make any corrections. For example, if you have gained weight, the air pressure would need to be changed.

Side Effects Of Using CPAP

The first few nights of using CPAP would get on your nerves. Many people feel CPAP extremely uncomfortable to wear. You may want to stop the treatment. What is advisable is to start off with low air pressure.

A great number of people who use CPAP have side effects. However, most of them have to do with the mask itself. For this, you need to select a mask which is comfortable and this prevents air pressure from leaking. With CPAP, the common side effects include:

- Nose Sores from wearing the device
- Chest muscles discomfort
- Congestion in your nasal area
- Dry or sore mouth
- Irritate eyes
- Nose and throat irritation
- Too much air pressure, therefore make it difficult for you to exhale
- Infections in your upper respiratory area

Adjusting the CPAP is perhaps the first thing to change. Seek advice from your sleep specialist or physician on how to do this. The moment you know how to do it, it would save you incredible amount of money as you wouldn't need to visit the specialist again and again.

There are also devices that would help you get more air in your throat. They can be adjusted and could be easily suited to fit your needs to ensure that air flows through your throat easily.

This device would change the air pressure while you are sleeping according to your needs. There isn't a push button as the adjustments are done automatically when you are deep asleep.

Using an oral appliance or mouthpiece is another great option if you find that CPAP doesn't work as well for you. It helps to keep your throat open so you can get as much air as possible. This is especially used for those who are dealing with a milder condition of sleep apnea.

Although CPAP is generally more effective than the oral appliance, the oral appliance is generally used by more people while they are asleep. This is because of the relative discomfort of using CPAP and the ease of using oral appliance.

Oral appliances open your throat. This is done by moving your lower jaw forward and would help your snoring and treat your sleep apnea situation. To get the oral appliance, ask your local dentist. You have to ensure that you get the right one and one you are comfortable with.

Do check with your dentist every half year after you start with it. After a year of wearing it, you could check with the dentist annually instead. This is to make sure that it is still comfortably and functioning well. At any time when you feel uncomfortable with it, seek your doctor instantly to ensure it is possibly adjusted.

Sleep Apnea Pillows

Some people get the right amount of sleep but still end up very tired during the day. This is because of their snoring, as snoring is a very serious medical issue. As such, a sleep apnea pillow can be used to cure it.

Sleep apnea pillows have been known to be very effective in treating sleep apnea in certain people. Before trying one, you need to know if your problem is that you are just snoring or if your snoring is because of your obstructive sleep apnea. However, sleep apnea pillows can help your snoring even if your condition isn't because of sleep apnea problems.

This special pillow is designed where the foam panels are elevated unlike normal pillows. This elevation would ensure that your head is slanted and improve the breathing pattern. This ensures that your breathing is regular and not interrupted.

A great number of sleep apnea pillows are made where they could be used in more than a single sleeping position. You can adjust them so you can sleep in the most comfortable sleeping position for you and provide quality support to ensure that you get a good night's sleep. Besides all these benefits, sleep apnea pillows also help:

- Open Blocked Airways, this ensures that your snoring and sleep apnea is relieved.
- Sleep Like A Baby
- Provides comfort and support to ensure that you have a good night's sleep
- Relieves you from chronic fatigue during the daytime

Many chronic snorers never use these kind of pillows and aren't keen to try them. Rather than that, they look to use sleeping pills. However, they end up being overly dependent on them. Medication isn't the proper alternative in assisting you with your sleep apnea or snoring. Try to stay away from medication, if possible.

Summary On Sleep Apnea

In this book, I have shared many ways of dealing with sleep apnea. Sleep apnea is a condition that has to be treated as early as possible. Below are some important points that you must know about sleep apnea.

- Obstructive sleep apnea is the most common form of sleep apnea.

- Sleep apnea is a very serious condition where your sleep is interrupted because of your breathing problem.

- Sleep apnea patients are known for being chronic snorers. As snoring is considered normal for certain people, some people don't even know that they have them.

- If you are chronically sleepy during the day, it may cause an accident.

- Your close family members can help to determine if you have sleep apnea. He/she can see if you are choking or gasping for air during your sleep.

- If you have too much weight, look to lose some weight. From there, maintain your weight.

- There are different treatments for sleep apnea. Your physician or sleep specialist would get the best treatment for you. This depends a lot on the seriousness of your condition.

- You shouldn't make fun of those people with sleep apnea.

- Look to cure sleep apnea immediately.
- Be on a lookout for children who have sleep apnea. They often have issues or other behavioral problems with the studies. Their self-esteem may also be affected.

Final Notes On Sleep Apnea

If diagnosed with sleep apnea, the conditions are not easily recognized. As such, many people go through their lives completely unaware of it. Someone may notice something wrong while you are asleep.

Just because you are snoring doesn't mean that you have this condition. However, many people who suffer from sleep apnea tend to be chronic snorers.

Therefore, the only way to decide if you have this condition is to do thorough examinations and sleep studies.

If someone close to you suspects that something is wrong with your sleeping pattern, you need to consult a physician as soon as you can. This early detection can be the big difference between treatment and getting a serious health issue. Don't ignore it.

Resource 1 - Sleep Apnea Exercises

A 20-min a day exercise program that help you cure sleep apnea from home...

In this guide, you have **18 step-by-step videos** that show you how to perform these exercises which are specially created to deal with SLEEP APNEA and a **52-Page illustrated manual**.

The manual includes these sections:

- Scientific studies backing up sleep apnea exercises

- **Daily tasks to keep your sleep apnea at a low level**
- Names and website addresses of speech language pathologists in the U.S. and U.K. who specialize in sleep apnea, and have agreed to list their contact details in my manual.
- **Names and contact details for obstructive sleep apnea support groups**
- MP3 (audio) recordings of the exercises that you can download and listen to on your iPod, iPhone, or MP3 device. (This is especially useful for the exercises that you'll want to do in front of the mirror)
- **Access to an online Members' Area, where you'll be able to download the manual, watch the videos, and get the bonuses!**

Go to this link to get this guide:

http://sleepapneaexercises.wellbeingvalley.com/

Resource 2 - Cure Sleep Apnea Without The Use of CPAP

Read the story about **how sleep apnea could kill you.** This <u>shocking</u> story tells how you **why you need to know all you need to know about CPAP**.

In this link, is a <u>FREE VIDEO</u> that you should definitely watch if you have SLEEP APNEA.

Head on to this link to watch it:

http://curesleepapnea.wellbeingvalley.com/